The
Handbook
For New Massage Therapist

By Daniella Whittle

Copyright

TABLE OF CONTENTS

Dedication

I am thankful for the many great instructors I have had and to every client that allowed me the opportunity to give them a massage. I am blessed to have a great family and amazing kids, who keep life exciting. Through them I have come to better understand my own philosophies, techniques and therapeutic touch.

I have dedicated this book to those who are making massage a career change, a hobby or are just interested in the world of all that massage therapy has to offer.

Preface

Are you new to massage therapy? Going to massage school?

Just graduate?

This is reference book written by a seasoned massage therapist. It will give you a jump-start into the practical world of massage therapy as a business and cut out years of learning by trial-and-error. It is designed exclusively to provide new massage therapist with a basic guide to long term success. It touches on key principles that will teach you exactly what elements matter most in retaining clients and divulge the best kept secrets in the business. Just by using a few simple tricks, you will be able to give an incredible massage that will eliminate even the most veteran competition!

Introduction

Do you have what it takes to make it in this business? Massage therapy is not just a job; it becomes a part of you! Massage is a discipline of your mind. You are putting aside yourself and giving to another. Before you touch a client you must answer the following prerequisite questions:

1. Will I leave the thoughts and emotions of my personal life at the door?

2. Will I focus and be present with this individual through the entire massage?

3. Will I give this client an amazing massage?

The answer to these questions should be a solid enthusiastic, "Yes"! Massage is highly interactive, in the sense that you are listening to the non verbal body language of your client at all times. Mastering this with each client is a daily practice. It is one of the first steps towards giving a massage that will have a memorable impact on your client.

Most massage therapists are paid per massage so you want to do what it takes to make the most out of your session. A successful massage session will achieve the following:

1. You met your client's expectations.

2. You up sold your service or/and sold retail products

3. The client rebooked with you.

If no one told you in massage school how important it is to be business savvy, I will lay it out for you. Massage therapist and business go hand in hand. You have to be good at both. There is no separating the two. You are now a business professional. You have to apply all the skills necessary to get the most from your time with your client. It requires individual growth, business sense, creativity, attention to detail and excellent interpersonal communication skills.

There are many dynamics at play when considering what it means to be a successful massage therapist. During your massage session with a client, you have a lot to accomplish! The critical moments that will make or break you will appear to roll together in one. This handbook breaks up your hour session and takes a look at each responsibility as a separate entity. Every detail and every element of your job needs to be looked at as its own skill. This is a great way to evaluate your strengths and weaknesses during your session. Maybe you are great at giving a massage but do not like sales? Or maybe you are not getting the best massage reviews but you are extremely knowledgeable in anatomy and have a passion for a certain type of massage? There is always somewhere to improve and it is easy to do if you just try something different with your next client. There is no shortage of opportunities to practice and get better!

You

The Massage Therapist

As a new massage therapist, you are the collective experience of your classroom training, hands on experience and who you are as person. If you are serious about making a living through massage therapy, you have to establish goals. What are your 3-month goals? Six months? One year? This is not a get rich quick job. It takes hard work, consistency, passion and self-care to weather through this business. It takes an enormous amount of giving of yourself and an unwavering sense of professionalism. That being said, it is an incredibly rewarding career that will change your life.

You Are Your Business

You are now your own business. Everything you do and say as a massage therapist is a reflection of your business model, from your clothes, to your handshake, to your business cards. Always be prepared for potential new clients. You are a reflection of your business. Be aware of how you are presenting yourself as you walk out the door. Carry business cards wherever you go and know your prices. Think of yourself as a walking billboard for your business.

Personal Evaluation

Massage therapists and clients build long-lasting relationships. How do you want to be seen? How do you cut out the competition? How would you evaluate your personal strengths and weaknesses? Does your business need improvements to make more money and bring in more clients? You have to evaluate yourself! You can ask your clients to fill out a personal feedback form of your work very similar to a Yelp review or ask an experienced massage therapist to give you an honest critique.

Pretend you are your own corporation. Your goal is to satisfy your customers, create great relations, make sure your clients are well taken care of and of course, make money. You have to be willing to learn, network and be consistent. At the end of the day, you are your most important asset to success.

Don't Sell Yourself Short

You are in business for yourself, and massage therapy is hard work. Offering your services too low in price means you will walk away being underpaid and burnt out. This is where your entrepreneurial skills and sales spirit will come into use! As massage therapists we are givers, we are empathetic, we are compassionate, but we need to survive too. We deserve to make a reasonable living, and there is nothing wrong with selling extra services or products. You are in control of what you make. It is important that you let go of the forty hour work week, eight hour day mentality.

Sales make an impact and every little bit helps. It could mean the difference between renting a house and buying a house. Wherever you work or plan to work, ask if you can sell your own products. Most employers will say yes, as long as it does not interfere or compete with their own retail products. When you highly recommend great products that you personally believe in, products sell themselves. There should always be a way you can make commission off products. Explore your options.

The Total Experience

The Working Environment

When you are working in a poor quality environment your work suffers. By poor quality environment, I mean bad management, substandard customer service, disorganization, low morale among workers, high drama, and unsafe or unsanitary conditions. I have worked for places like this and my suggestion is to find another place to work ASAP. Quality businesses and management will strive to maintain balance, appreciate their employees, have high customer service integrity and will usually have outstanding reviews. Do not settle for less! If you are new in the industry and have no references yet, I would suggest working for a high-end spa whose reputation precedes them. At the very least, you can check out the competition and experience what the best means for you on the receiving end of a massage. You can emulate that quality of service in your practice. If you want to be the best, only work for and work with the best.

Décor

Your client will begin to judge their ability relax the moment they enter your physical space. A key point to remember is, "Like often attracts like". For example, if your massage space is decked out in crystals, heavy incense, and aura lights, then of course you are going to attract more of a metaphysical crowd. On the opposite end of the spectrum, if your room is set up like a doctor's office, that will also attract a different type of clientele. So my advice before you do any decorating is to take your time and think about what type of massage therapist you are. Are you more on the ethereal side, neutral and spa-like or more of a medical therapist? Once you have decided on your décor ask yourself, "What clientele am I attracting? What clientele may I be repelling? Does my décor, project me as the massage therapist?" Visit other salons or massage clinics and look online. Get an idea of what will work for you. You're creating the experience! Creating a space that will reflect you takes thought and preplanning. It also takes money to do all this and it is best to narrow down exactly what you want before you buy anything related to your business.

If you are working for someone else, you should do everything you can to personalize the room and stand out from the crowd. You may be working for a spa or office where the decorative aspect will be taken care of. You should bring in items that will give your room a personal touch. The same thought still applies! Any décor you bring is still a reflection of your business and you as a massage therapist. Choose wisely.

Smell

Smell is everything! When your client walks in, do you want them to smell massage oils? Incense? Cleaning products? Nothing? Fresh scent? Whatever the smell you choose, keep it consistent. We all know what walking into a pizza joint smells like with our eyes closed. You want your repeat clients to link the smell of your room to your massage with their eyes closed. As your repeat clients walk in, the familiar smell will subconsciously start training their mind and body to relax. I have found many clients prefer no heavy scents in the air, unless they willingly choose it as a cream or oil during their massage. People are very sensitive to smells as well as any scented fragrance you wear! Always check in with your client and keep a note on what your client likes or does not like.

That being said, on a side note, if you do not shower regularly or wear deodorant and think you don't ever smell, you are wrong. That's just you getting used to it. After multiple massages you will smell! This can deter clients and puts those who work with you in an awkward position to speak to you about your hygiene. We all get sweaty and hot during a massage! If you need to reapply deodorant or wipe down after a massage, then do it. You can always ask a fellow massage therapist if you smell. Carry towels, wipes or whatever you need, to keep yourself fresh. Another common complaint is bad breath. We do not want our fingers and breathe to smell like the tuna and onion sandwich we just had for lunch. Smell is powerfully linked to memory and we only want our clients to remember the fresh smell of aromatherapy, lotions and oils during the massage, not our body odor.

Cleanliness

Wash your hands before you ever touch a client's body. If the sink is out of the room, let them know that you have just washed your hands when you re-enter the room to give them a massage. The cleanliness of your hands might not be on every clients mind, but those clients who are very particular about germs and observant will take note that you didn't wash your hands. Some clients may walk right out of the massage room because you touched them without washing your hands. It is better to be sure and address hand washing in some way before each massage begins. Be mindful of oil and lotion that splatter on ground because it will gleam against any flooring, even in the dimmest of light. Your client will notice everything! And everything counts when it comes to retaining your client and a getting positive review. Disinfect all bottles, massage equipment and surfaces in your space. You may be working on the fourth client of the day, but you still want to make each client feel as though they are the first in the room. Clients don't want to enter a room that looks like the sheets were carelessly thrown on the massage table. Your supplies on the counter should not have that unorganized, greasy, slick look from your last massage. Always come prepared with hand sanitizer, disinfectant spray, water, towels or anything you need to do a swift and thorough clean-up job in between clients. Take care to fix the room before each client.

Music

Create a peaceful setting for yourself and for your client. Have options! For repeat clients you can create their own personal playlist or let them know they can bring in their own music. If you have the ability to change the music playing, always ask your client their preference. Not all clients relax to Native American music with flutes and chants. For some, it's Jack Johnson, Pink Floyd and Elvis. So be open-minded to all music and give your clients the option to choose their music for a more personalized experience.

Lights

Lights set the stage, so to speak, and create an experience. What kind of lighting do you like? A bright natural light or dark and dim lights? Candles? Lamps? Projected wall lights? The lighting should be consistent with your décor and business model. You can go dim and spa-like or have an array of trace lighting for an ethereal set up. A fluorescent, brighter, or natural window light set up, could be for a clinical or neutral atmosphere. Keep in mind, some clients may not be able to see in dim settings. Always have bright light available just in case. Some people are not comfortable with the light turned down low, and others would prefer the least light possible. No matter what kind of light set up you have, always maintain awareness of your clients' needs. Ask during the initial consultation if they are comfortable with the lighting.

Consultation

Project Relaxation

During the consultation, you should maintain a positive, calm nature. Begin to lower your voice, talk a little slower, be more breathy, and use that sort of rock a baby to sleep talk, if you need to. There are many clients who are extremely high strung, loud, and have no awareness yet that they are in a quiet, serene atmosphere. By using a slower, calmer tone when speaking to the client, you are facilitating the reason why they have come to see you today. Usually, clients will follow your lead once you begin to lower your voice. Keep in mind that any interaction with them should always be about creating a relaxing environment. They are paying you for a massage that should be a relaxing, safe, personal break from the high stress environment outside of the walls of your room or spa.

Notes

Yes, we all learned about S.O.A.P notes! In the real world, you are not going to be taking detailed notes on every client unless you work for yourself, a chiropractor, doctor or a medical facility where insurance billing may be involved. Regardless, at any facility, clients receiving a service should have to fill out a waiver and or medical information card which allow them to state any conditions that might be a contraindication for massage. You should always have access to these records and request to see them on every new client.

Once your client enters your room, you have to follow up with a verbal consultation! Any extra relevant information you get, should be put in your notes. Key examples are injuries, pregnancy, open cuts, scarring, rashes, arthritis, recent surgeries, etc. You also need to ask if there is a specific area they would like you to spend more time on or avoid completely. Reiterate and confirm the type of massage they are requesting. More often than not, a client's memory of their pain or other issues will be triggered during their massage as you pass over certain body parts. Put that information in their notes as well. You can take notes on any client. It is your right and in your best interest to do so. If you are taking notes, make your questions count and be very specific about all details. You can also use your intake form as a cheat sheet during your consultation if you need practice.

C.O.A.T. (Communicate=Observe, Ask, Tone)

In other words, while doing your initial consultation with your client, you should be observing their nonverbal body language, asking questions and using the proper tone when speaking to them.

Observe: What's the client's age range? Did they come in solo, with a group or as a couple? What kind of pressure did they give you in their hand shake? What is their walking speed? How do they walk? What day, and what time of day did they come in? How are they dressed? Did they come in sweats or are they dressed to go out? Is their hair done perfectly? Do they have jewelry on? Are they male or female? This gets your wheels turning on what to address during your consultation and to help better serve your clients during their massage. For example, an elderly lady with stiff curls, lots of jewelry who limps and walks unsteadily to your massage room might need, the lights in the room brighter, the table lowered, extra pillows to get comfortable and a little extra time to get undressed and dressed. As part of your consultation, you already know you will have to address possible injuries, stiffness, maybe arthritis and areas to avoid. You need to ask her to take off the jewelry and find out whether or not she would like you to avoid her hair.

Now at the other end of the spectrum, you have a fast walking male in his 30's that comes in wearing sweats and a T-shirt, looks physically fit, and stares at the table as you speak to him. He has already begun to take his watch and shirt off, while giving you short responses to your consultation questions. These kinds of clients have a need to get on the table and relax, right away. I will say, "Ok, face down and I will be right back," and walk out. His body language is telling me he wants on the table, now! I will check his initial paperwork to see if he gave any indication that he was other than, perfectly healthy. When I reenter the room I will then proceed with my consultation. A young fit guy would, quite possibly have had a major surgery or injury so I would ask, right away about injuries and then finish up with a couple more brief questions. Do not force talk, except for questions pertinent to the health and well-being of you or your client. Follow your client's lead and respect what his/her non-verbal body language is saying. As a massage therapist, the more observant you become the better you will serve your clients. You need to observe everything and go with flow of your client.

Ask: If your client says, their back is sore, you say where? Why? Their toenail fell off?   Which foot and which toe. Ask questions! Be as specific as possible and hone in on exactly what and where they are talking about.

Tone: The tone of voice will often convey more meaning than words. I will hear clients say in an exhausted manner, "I am really stressed out from work" and in the same sentence say, "I really like deep work and you can press as hard you want". Clients have no concept of their therapist's ability to apply pressure, just as we have no concept of what the best pressure for them is before we touch our clients and do a pressure check. You have to make sense of what the client tells you because pressing too hard and or going too deep may not actually relax them. In most cases, unless your client has an injury, is an athlete or uses their body repetitively for work, the kind of pressure being requesting will not be necessary. More often than not, the client's first initial reaction and the tone of their voice will tell you the most about what kind pressure and massage they need.

Stay On Point

If you are not already experienced in consultations, it doesn't take long to get comfortable with them and become a pro. If the conversation starts getting lengthy and leads into other areas that have nothing to do with the specific consultation, then you need to take charge and lead them back to the massage at hand. Stick to the point as much as possible. If you can't find your way out of the conversation, you can interject by looking at the clock and then say, "Oh, it's two minutes past the hour. I want to give you as much time as possible on the table, so I am going to step out and let you get changed". You can lead with a distraction, such as to double check if they need to use the restroom and then lead with your exit speech. Just stay on point during the consultation and make sure any interruption is as graceful as possible and only to get back on topic.

Accommodations

Before you leave the room, let your clients know where to put their things, where the tissues, wipes, mints and water are. Let them know you have pillows if they need them, and you will adjust everything when you come back into the room. Try to address all questions that you think they might have. Make them feel welcome and comfortable, as if they are your royal guest. Be patient and caring to all needs during the course of your entire interaction. Clients love the royal treatment in care, compassion and sensitivity to their needs.

The Zone

Get There

If you, the therapist aren't relaxed, not one of your clients will be. Develop a routine that gets you into your massage zone. It could be exercise, humming, chanting or listening to your favorite music. Do what works for you. What works for me is setting my room up, the table, the lights and actually doing the massage. As massage therapist, we are not always on massage-flow status. We need to put in a little effort in order to give a great massage! You must find the balance in yourself to create a pure, open space for that client. I call it, going into "The Zone".

This can be a challenge, considering the types of stress life throws our way. If you booked four massages for the day, that is four hours of silence. Do not put yourself on auto pilot and space out. You will be doing poor quality work and there is no *giving* involved. You still have to maintain presence and awareness. That is your duty and part of your job description. You are not serving your client by tuning into your own world for the hour.

Confidence

This is a success secret! Your confidence is displayed in your initial handshake, eye contact, communication and in your belief that you can give the best massage. Not just the best, but a memorable massage experience. You have to believe with every fiber, thought and vibration in your body that you can set the space to give your client a great massage. It's about being in "The Zone" with your client and knowing that you gave 110 percent to that individual during their whole massage. Just by mastering the simple step of being present, aware, and completely in tune to your client you will be giving your clients the best you. There can be no doubt in your mind that you will give your client the absolute most relaxing, healing, warming, gooey, melty, stuck to the table massage ever! YOU HAVE TO BELIEVE IT, period!! There is no other option. Your client is coming to you for a service, an experience, a pain reliever, a treatment, a break from the daily grind. You have to believe that you are present in that moment, with that person to facilitate their needs and go above and beyond their expectations. You are the massage therapist. You are in your element, and you chose this life, this career, this path which has landed you in this massage room with this client, now! YOU MUST BELIEVE there is a reason for your connection with this person and it is meant to do the ultimate good for their wellbeing. You must do quality work every single time you put your hands on a client. If you have trouble believing this strongly in your work, than find a way to get there. It comes from within.

The Massage

Professionalism

When you greet clients for their massage, use your best etiquette, open all doors and give them a smile. From your client's perspective, you should not have a care in the world. It's all about them during their session. They are coming in to receive, relax, relieve and renew. Do not ever tell a first- time client anything about your personal life that would cause them to sympathize or feel bad for you. Do not vent to them! Your first job is to retain that client and allow him/her to focus on themselves and their body, not their stresses and not your stress. You also, don't want your repeat clients to go to another massage therapist so they can relax, because you have now become friends with this person and you talk and play catch up during their massage. You want their session to be exactly what a massage is designed for, every single time they come to see you. Always maintain an awareness of the service they are paying for and the level of professionalism you need to maintain at all times. It's still your business and your clients are clients! Respect that boundary. If you want to make money and keep your clients, maintain your professionalism!

Comfort-Ability

There are many changes going on in a person's body during a massage, some of which include temperature, drainage, possible itching, twitching, and a wide variety of emotions. At any time your client could need to stretch, adjust the head rest, blow their nose, turn, require an extra pillow or use the restroom. Be patient and courteous to all their needs while giving them a massage. Your job is to check in verbally as well as to observe the client's body language so you can adjust to their needs for those clients who will not freely tell you if they are uncomfortable. It is your ability to be attentive to your clients during the massage that will keep them comfortable. If you are not mindful of their comfort you will not get return clients.

Relaxation=Receiving

GET YOUR CLIENT TO RELAX. This is the most fundamental objective during a massage. This is the gateway that allows your client to receive and accept your massage. Massage is truly a give and receive exercise. Not all clients know how to receive the full benefit of your massage and it is your job to find a way to help them do that.

 With the stress of today's world, an hour massage never seems like enough time for clients to really soak into your table and totally relax. During the massage, the average time to start feeling a difference in a person's tissue is about twenty minutes. That's why, whatever you can do to begin to relax your client as soon as they walk through the door, the easier your work will be and the better for your client. Your work is useless if a person cannot relax during the massage. Be sensitive to the fact that relaxation is very individualized. There are those clients who will accept your massage and melt right into the table. They are great receivers, who will breathe into each massage stroke. That is when you can give your best massage. Then, there are those who chatter the whole time, speak with their hands, tighten up every muscle when they talk and the word relax is foreign to them. It's your job to help each client relax based on what is right for the type of client you are working with.

Pain or Tension

Always check in with your client and get a doctor's note before working on anyone with a new injury, who is post-surgery, has cancer or anything you may physically see that looks like it may be a contraindication for massage. Stay away from anything that is swollen, bruised, has medical dressing, rashes, oozing fluid, scabbing and anything other than normal healthy skin. Do not be afraid to ask questions and say "No," you will not work the area without a doctor's note or just a straight "No, I cannot give you a massage today because..". Of course, be very polite about it. Take extreme caution and use the proper procedures when dealing with medical conditions. Just know that you are in control of your session. Do not let clients bully you to work areas that you need a doctor's note for. When there is pain involved, clients tend to be short tempered and very demanding.

When we are in pain from tense and overworked muscles, there's is nothing better than somebody touching those sore areas and relieving the pain right away. Just the pressure is satisfying! The same is true with your clients. As a massage therapist you may know that your client's pain may be coming from another area, or that the area needs to be warmed up before getting in deeper. Clients who request a full body massage and have pain will rarely allow you the time to get to their hot spots on your own, during the course of their full body massage. You can recognize clients like this right away, because they will say, "That's the spot," several times, as you keep grazing over the area during the first couple minutes of massage, or they will swing their arm up and lead you back to area by pointing to the spot again. The warm up is like a teaser. Once you gather that you are working on a client like this, do an initial 3-5 minutes of massage on their problem spot, and then rework it however you want and however many times you want as you go through the body massage. This strategy gives the client that "AWW" feeling right away. It is just enough to satisfy your client so they can relax and enjoy the rest of their massage. Otherwise, they spend the whole massage wondering when you are going to get to their hot spots and will not be able to relax.

Pressure Check

It doesn't matter how long you have been in the business, you should always do a pressure check. Everybody is different! Just when you think you have mastered the art of pressure, there is always another client to tell you it's too deep, too light or that a certain spot hurts when you massage the area. A verbal pressure check is a must. You should never make an assumption about what the best pressure is in any area of your client's body, even if you are a skilled practitioner. Deeper pressure doesn't always mean or equate to feeling better. We are working with the brain first! Our bodies naturally want to feel safe and relaxed. The moment a deep pressure is applied on the body, the more likely your clients are going to tense up. You need to work your way into deep pressure if it is a true deep tissue massage. Keep in mind that a normal, healthy body is not going to need massive amounts of elbow and finger pressure over their entire body to get their muscles to relax.

There is a little thing called "Stress," that can tighten the back, creep up and squeeze the neck to make its constant presence known. It is not a muscular condition; it is a state of mind! Any pain associated with stress is just stress. It's not a true physical injury yet. Your observation skills are essential to picking up on what is really going on with your client.

One of the first long-term clients I had on a weekly basis was always tight. His back was like a cement wall. I constantly used deep pressure on him. It seemed as though my pressure was never deep enough and I could never break through that barrier. Well, I didn't see him for about a month, which was weird because he was a steady client. When he rebooked and then came in for his appointment, I will never forget what it felt like when I put my hands on his back, for the first time in over a month. I gasped, and asked him, "What happened? This is incredible! Your back is bouncy and loose?" His muscles felt like warm, healthy putty that was pliable and easy to glide through. I could not believe it. All the weeks of hard strenuous massages and now, viola! It was like touching a completely different body. So when I asked what happened, he told me that he quit his job! That is when it hit me. All the weeks of hard work, deep tissue and stretching had no impact on him because it was all mental stress. And the best thing I could have been doing for him was actually giving him a relaxing, pampering massage experience when he came in. I could have easily recognized that he needed a different kind of massage. I could have recommended a service that would have actually benefited him. Could have, would have, and should have, but too late. So I learned my lesson.

My rule of thumb on pressure is to never assume that you know what pressure feels right for your client, and never assume that the pressure that feels right for your client is actually what is going to benefit them. We have to focus in and use all of our skills and intuition to give the client the right massage. There is not one perfect recipe for pressure that will work every single time with any client, or even repeat clients. It's about what works on this day, now, for this client on the table. If you have a regular client and nothing you're doing is working, it is probably a good sign that you need to try something different. Find what actually works to relax your client. You can always make suggestions as to the type of massage you recommend for them and why, but do not be pushy. Be flexible with your clients and give them the knowledge so they can make a more informed decision on the type of massage or service they book next.

Clients

First-Time-Ever Massage

When you greet your client, act like getting a massage is the most natural and normal everyday occurrence. No awkward silence. The more at ease you make your client feel, the better. Explain to them how to get on the table, their options for clothing and what they may experience during and after the massage. Let them know you will be there to get anything they need. Give them tips on how to relax their body. A young client or just a first-timer that is not quite comfortable with massage are great examples of the kinds of clients you can make conversation with during the massage. It will likely allow them to relax a little bit more. Make sure your client is draped tightly at all times and explain any movement or exposure when it comes to the sheet before you do it. Keep your clients at ease by answering their anticipated questions. You are telling them what to expect so there are no surprises, helping them to feel comfortable.

You are giving this person a massage for the very first time. This is a blessing! You need to make sure their experience is great, and they will want to come back for another. It's like spreading the word of massage through each client. Be grateful that you are the one giving them their first massage and that you are creating future business for yourself and for all massage therapists.

The First-Time Client

Do not let a first-time client idly go through your massage without making an impression. Educate your clients on what you do and the services you offer. Always recommend 90 minute massages for those who need it. An hour is just not enough for most people. Let your client know how often they should get a massage and establish repeat bookings right away. Get out your calendar and schedule your client to receive another massage. Get them on a routine and make massage a part of their lives. If they don't reschedule with you right away, wait a couple of weeks, call them back and offer a special deal. Make an impression! Building a repeat client from a first time client is your goal. This is your bread and butter and what makes your business grow. Establishing a repeat client is a success!

Repeat Clients

The experience of your massage is already implanted in a repeat client's mind. It starts from the moment they decide they are going to rebook. For these clients, every massage session with you has to meet their expectations of your work or exceed the level of service from their previous experience. This is when delivering only your personal best comes into play and why being consistent in your work is so crucial. If you can do this, then you have a client for life. Rebook their appointment right away. Let them know what changes you felt on their body, if anything, from when you worked on them last. Let them know about any upcoming specials you have, and as always, have retail products available.

Repeat clients love when you experiment new techniques on them. They are great guinea pigs. If you are always growing as a therapist and are willing to give great work every single time, clients will follow you and they will refer you to everybody they know. Before you know it, you will be working on all their family members and friends. That is how your business will start to grow.

The Wrap Up

Recommendations

You are not a medical professional and have no idea what a person's true medical condition or history may be. You are not a nutritionist either. Do not recommend, "A lot of water to clear the toxins," after the massage. You have no idea if your client is taking medication or has a medical condition in which a lot of water would make them sick or cause death. A perfect example of what to say at the end of the conversation with your client is "Thank you so much for coming in! Enjoy your day, relax and I will see you next time". We can get in a lot of trouble for recommending anything outside of our scope of practice. So I say, keep it brief and simple unless backed up by a medical professional.

The only recommendations I give to my clients are other services I offer or other people I refer. Anything else I say to a client is regarding what I felt during the massage. I will start with the words, "I noticed". For example, "I noticed that your left side is tighter than the right". Maybe they carry their purse on their left arm? There could be numerous reasons for why the left side is tighter. Share just enough, to make them aware of what you felt to get their own wheels turning. If I feel a lump or solid fatty tissue during the massage, I will say, "What is this?" If they did not already know it was there, it is now brought to their attention. I am not in any way putting a name to it or telling them to go to the doctor. I am simply stating what I noticed.

You also do not want to stress out your clients during their massage, so use your best judgment. Our gift and scope of practice is bringing your clients to a deeper awareness of their bodies through touch. Clients have free reign to do with that what they will, without your diagnosis or recommendations which may be wrong. Use caution with what you say because clients will ask you what to do, what you recommend and what you think. You have to be somewhat tactical in your response.

On The Clock

Do not get in the habit of talking with clients for a long time, after your massage, even if you have time, because that will be expected of you every time. Clients will look forward to that! Of course, you will have the occasional gab when you have time, but when you are busy, pay your respects to the client, take care of business and then get ready for your next appointment. You are always in control of actively managing your time on the clock.

Long Term Success

Avoid Burnout/Injury

All too often massage therapists sell their souls for $12 a massage at six-plus clients a day, for years on end. Massage therapy has gone corporate and we can work 40 hours a week for a standard hourly pay. Massage therapists are not meant to do mass massages and be structured like a standard job. Get out of that mindset if this is you. This is an easy way to get injured. Granted, for new therapists in the business, it is a great way to gain experience. It is not something to do long term. This is how injuries happen and why many massage therapists have to change careers.

Massage therapists give and give. We give as a part of our work. When you are over-worked at work and over worked in your personal life. You will get burned out! You need to receive as well. Getting regular massages, stretching and exercise will help balance your work and personal life when you are burning the candle at both ends. Taking care of your mind and body is extremely important in this business, since it is the tool we use for our work.

Energy

Massage is an energetic interaction. It can give you energy and drain you. The type of drain I am talking about will feel like you spent a 12-hour day walking in the scorching sun. It is a deep, energetic drain. You have to block yourself from taking on your client's energy or giving your energy to them. You can easily take your client's injuries and emotions home with you. Those who practice Reiki or do other types of energy work, will have a head start on how to protect themselves. If you are new in the field, you will have to learn how to manage this energy exchange and use it to your advantage to help your client. There are many books and online sources that can lead you in the right direction.

Positive attitude

You are going to be sore and tired at times, but every massage you give has to be quality and you have to maintain that positive spirit with each client for success. This comes from the inner source that brought you to do massage in the first place-the inner spirit of healing and caring. You are interacting with people on a very personal level and your attitude will be apparent in your work.

41

Living a positive lifestyle consistent with being a massage therapist

is really helpful for making massage therapy a long term career, love

and passion.

Hands on Massage Tips

Massage Technique

If you are a new massage therapist, over time you will develop an arsenal of skills in your tool bag. So not to worry! THE TRUTH IS- You do not need to have any advanced techniques to give a client an unforgettable massage. Human touch is vital to our growth and development. It feels great when your significant other pushes on your sore feet or sore back even though they have no professional training. Touch feels good for most people! All you need is presence, confidence, a consistent flow and a sense of being in tune with your client.

Fresh out of school I was getting raves by clients who had gotten massages all over the world. It made me think-why? It was certainly not technique, in comparison to a more veteran masseuse. So what am I doing right? I had acquired maybe a total of 6 or 7 massage moves that I used consistently. Does technique have to be there to give that client a wonderful massage or even the best massage they have ever had? The answer is no. You do not need to know any fancy moves to get clients and keep clients!

Flow

All you need is flow! This is where you can cut out and eliminate the more veteran competition. Flow has a natural rhythm, energy and dynamic movement to it. Just like babies, people love to be rocked and swayed to a natural rhythm that will put them to sleep. People are drawn to music, dance and any art that makes us feel a sense of release. A good massage therapist can provide this flow for their client.

A massage that has flow means one movement goes right into another. Your massage moves should overlap and complement each other without choppy movements into an unexpected part of the body. This allows the client's body to relax, unwind and let go. So much about any type of massage is allowing the client to relax and feel completely comfortable.

Accommodations

By accommodations I mean anything that your client would possibly need. This includes, wipes for sensitive skin, tissues, essential oils, sugar free and regular mints, a robe and slippers to throw on in case they need to use the restroom, heating pad, heater, extra blankets, pillows of all shapes and sizes, extra towels to wipe off oil if needed, trash can, mirror, water bottle with a business sticker, samples of your products with a business sticker, anatomy books, etc. If you are prepared for any possible need your client may have during the massage, the more professional you appear and the more your client takes comfort in knowing you have everything they need to feel safe, secure and taken care of.

Presentation

Thoroughly prepare your room in an orderly and presentable, clean appearance after each massage. Your room is an extension of your massage and a reflection of who you are. Fold your sheets a special way on the table that looks inviting, organize your bottles and creams so everything faces forward and is perfect. Presentation is not everything but it could count for a lot when you are competing for business with the other massage therapists in the area.

Be Consistent

Show up for your clients! Try not to reschedule your appointments. Your reputation will follow you. If you are being consistent on every level of your business, you will become the total embodiment of your work and a true professional. We want

massages to be seen as part of the health and wellness industry.

Anything you can do to give some credibility to our industry when

working with clients the better for the massage therapist community.

We represent each other!

Be Thorough

During your massage, leave no muscle untouched. Treat

every muscle as if it is its own unit. Think of it like tracing the

outline of each individual strand of muscle. Follow the muscles,

follow bones and use them to guide your fingers and hands. Do not

be afraid to move the sheets. Give a good, solid, complete massage.

Do not let your client walk away unsatisfied.

Be Creative

Can you name ten things that set you apart from the other

therapists? Switch things up! Use massage tools or incorporate them.

Practice what you learn in your continuing-education classes.

Customize your session and don't do the same cookie-cutter

massage for each client. Keep your clients guessing and ask for feedback. Be ever evolving as a therapist. Do not get stuck in a rut! Look for inspiration and fresh ideas for your business.

Money

Keep your massage quality consistent. Always up sell your services, offer retail products, packages and gift certificates. Realize that you are in the business of sales as well as being an incredibly awesome massage therapist! In order to make money long term, you have to be passionate about your work and charge what you are worth, within reason. Plan for your future and think of massage therapy as a career, a choice and a passion, not a job where you are limited to the same paycheck every week.

Last But Not Least

In massage school you learn anatomy and physiology, massage styles and techniques. You become aware of the power of therapeutic touch and what it means to give, receive and maintain balance. Then, as a working professional that knowledge is put to use in practical application. In the working environment you get a sense of your strengths and weaknesses. This is when you begin to develop into our own skin as a massage therapist. This process is known as the mind, body and spirit connection to your work.

There is no one right way to fully develop your skills. Finding your own path and developing your sense of what works for you, is part of the grand experience that creates an everlasting bond and love for massage therapy. It is about finding, "The best massage therapist in you". It is ever evolving!

New therapist, be adventurous! Find your niche in the massage world. What we do is help, heal and give a deeply needed service to a society with busy and stressful lives. Our work matters and is meaningful. Massage is a skill and an art you will have for life .You can offer help to anyone at any time. This is a career that is challenging, rewarding and relaxing! If you have a passion for

giving massages and helping others, you will go far.

 Good luck to you on your journey,

From one massage therapist to another-

Biography

I began my journey right out of high school in sunny San Diego. I signed up for a 1000 hour holistic program where I was able to receive certifications in a number of different specialties. Part of the course hours was a required 110 hours of massage. I remember thinking to myself, I don't want to rub lotion all over people, annoyed that I had to spend so many hours doing this. That statement makes me laugh now because I obviously had no idea about the importance, history and the powerful effect massage would have on me later in life. So I opted for 110 hour non-lotion, clothed course. I fell in love! From then on, I took every possible massage class I could get my hands on, literally!

I worked in many different settings, starting out at my school clinic, going to client's houses, spas, chiropractors and volunteering for events and marathons. I loved the fact that I was not stuck with one employer and one job. I could work in five different places five days of the week, if I wanted. I also loved being around like-minded individuals, who also practiced massage or were in the health and wellness industry. We share a common bond and understanding for healing and helping others.

When I started out as a massage therapist, I knew I was going to have to hustle. I knew clients were not going to just come to me. I was fortunate enough to start working at my school clinic which gave me plenty of clientele. At that time, I believe the charge for a massage was around $20 or $25. Over the next couple of years I took many more classes and worked in different settings. This is where I learned what the best means for me as a massage therapist. The best way to learn sometimes is by trial-and-error and exposure to different working environments. It became a personal challenge. I wanted my clients to remember my massage the next time they needed one.

I have never had a bad experience as a massage therapist! I found early on that I had to be completely comfortable with myself, know my own boundaries, and respect the boundaries and level of modesty of my clients. Ultimately, I take comfort in knowing that I have full control of any situation. I have always strongly believed my work is a reflection of myself and the massage therapist community as a whole. I feel it's my responsibility to reflect the highest integrity and professionalism when working with clients. I made my mind up right away that any experience with a new client will be guided by unwavering professionalism and an endless journey to make our work respected and credible in the health and wellness industry.

During my career I have been married and have had kids. I practice massage on my kids and in return they are just as excited to give me a massage. How awesome is that; a bunch of little feet smashing my back! It's a great give and receive exercise to do with the children.

I have been practicing massage since 2001, and I still to this day love what I do. I feel deeply that massage is a part of my life and my spirit. This skill is something I can do anytime, with just my hands. I am blessed I have a skill I can use to help people. It is a beautiful world with massages in it!

www.ingramcontent.com/pod-product-compliance
Lightning Source LLC
Chambersburg PA
CBHW050823290526
45792CB00001B/231